HOW TO TELL YOUR CHILD THEY HAVE CANCER

How to Tell Your Child They Have Cancer

and how to fight it...

JOHN H. SWINFORD III

IngramSpark

ACKNOWLEDGEMENT

Publisher: IngramSparks

Influencers:

    Dr. Melvin Dyster

    Dr. Daniel M. Green

    Dr. Martin L. Brecher

    My Mother – at the age of 26, faced with a child diagnosed with Stage 4 Burkitt lymphoma

    Roswell Park Cancer Institute; now Roswell Park Comprehensive Cancer Center

Contributor: ChatGPT Artificial Intelligence
Photos provided by: PNGWING

PRELUDE

First, my condolences, because if you are buying this book, your child or someone you know has a child with cancer. There are no words of sorrow that can be expressed. There are however words to encourage the fight and provide a shining light.

To a parent of a child with cancer, here are some words of hope and caring:

> Even in the face of such a challenging situation, remember that hope can be a powerful force. Stay strong and believe in your child's resilience and the possibility of healing.

> Your love and care for your child are extraordinary. Your unwavering support will be a source of strength for both of you throughout this journey.

> While it may feel overwhelming at times, remember that you are not alone. Countless people are rooting for your child's recovery, and we will walk this path alongside you.

Every day, medical research and advancements are being made to improve treatments and outcomes. Have faith in the expertise of the medical team, and remember that there are new possibilities and options to explore.

Your child's spirit and determination will serve as an inspiration to others. Their bravery and resilience are remarkable, and they have a community of people who believe in their ability to overcome this challenge.

Amidst the difficulties, find moments of joy and cherish them. Celebrate small victories, lean on the support of loved ones, and create precious memories that will strengthen your bond as a family.

Know that it's okay to have moments of doubt or vulnerability. Taking care of yourself emotionally and physically is crucial during this time. Lean on your support network, seek counseling if needed, and practice self-care to maintain your well-being.

While the road ahead may be long and arduous, hold onto the possibility of a brighter future. With advancements in medicine and the power of love and determination, there is always hope for better days."

~ 1 ~

HOW TO TELL YOUR CHILD

Telling a child about their cancer diagnosis and explaining how to fight cancer can be an extremely delicate and challenging conversation. Remember to use gentle and age-appropriate language while conveying the necessary information. Here are some suggestions for how to approach it with and the right words to use:

Choose an appropriate setting: Find a quiet and comfortable environment where the child feels safe and secure. Minimize distractions and ensure privacy to allow for an open and honest conversation. Use a hopeful and loving tone: Throughout the conversation, maintain a calm and loving tone. Reiterate your love for the child and your commitment to being there for them every step of the way.

Start with empathy and reassurance: Begin

the conversation by expressing your love and support for the child. Let them know that you care about them deeply and that you are there to support them throughout their journey.

Use simple and age-appropriate language: Tailor your explanation to the child's age and level of understanding. Be clear and concise using words and concepts that they can grasp without overwhelming them. Avoid using medical jargon and complicated terminology. Be honest, but also provide information in a way that they can comprehend.

Be calm and reassuring: Stay composed during the conversation and maintain a calm and reassuring demeanor. Children take cues from adults, so your calmness can help alleviate their anxiety. Make it clear to the child that having cancer is not their fault. Explain that cancer can happen to anyone, and it's not because of something they did or didn't do.

Explain the diagnosis gently: Use phrases like "there's something in your body that needs special attention" or "the doctors found some cells that need to be treated." Provide a basic explanation of cancer as an illness where the body's cells are not behaving the way they should. Let the child know that cancer is a disease, and the medical team will work to fight it.

Highlight the importance of treatment: Let the child know that there are special doctors and nurses who are experts at treating cancer. Assure them that the medical team will work together to help them get better. Explain that the treatment may involve medications, surgeries, or other procedures that will help them get better.

Emphasize their role in fighting cancer: Empower the child by explaining that they have an important role to play in fighting cancer. Encourage them to be brave, resilient, and emphasize that they are not alone. Assure them that they have the support of their family, medical team, and other loved ones.

Address possible side effects: Explain that the treatments they will receive may cause some changes in their body, such as hair loss, feeling tired, or changes in appetite. Assure them that these side effects are temporary and that the doctors will help manage them.

Address their emotions and concerns: Give the child an opportunity to express their feelings and concerns. Acknowledge their emotions, whether it's fear, sadness, anger, or confusion. Let them know that it's normal to have these feelings and that it's okay to talk about them.

Provide hope and optimism: While being honest about the challenges it's essential to be honest, it's also crucial to instill hope and optimism. Explain that many children have successfully fought cancer and that the treatment is designed to help them get better. Reinforce the idea that there is a chance for recovery and a return to a normal life.

Encourage questions, emotions, ongoing open communication: Let the child know that it's okay to feel scared, sad, or angry about the diagnosis. Let the child know that they can ask questions at any time. Encourage them to express any concerns or uncertainties they may have. Assure them that you are there to answer honestly and support them through their journey. Be prepared to provide ongoing support and reassurance as they navigate their cancer journey.

Offer ongoing support: Reassure the child that they are not alone and that they have a network of support, including their family, friends, and healthcare team. Let them know that they can lean on these people for emotional support, assistance, and any help they may need. Beware of available support resources, such as child life specialists, support groups, and counseling services. These resources can help them cope with the emotional and practical challenges they may encounter.

Involve the medical team: Reassure the child that they will have a dedicated team of doctors, nurses, and healthcare professionals who specialize in treating children with cancer. Emphasize that these professionals will be there to guide and support them throughout the treatment process.

Remember, each child is unique, and the conversation should be tailored to their specific needs and understanding. It may be helpful to consult with a child life specialist or a healthcare professional experienced in pediatric oncology to guide you through this conversation.

~ 2 ~

I HAVE SOMETHING TO TELL YOU

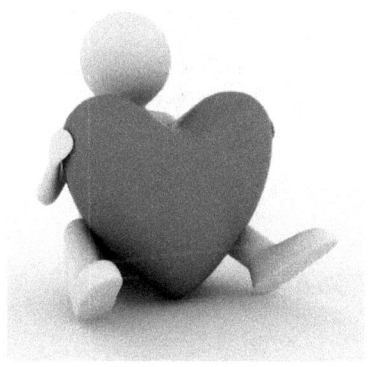

In your heart, a love so true,
Know that we'll always be here for you.
Through thick and thin, come what may,
Our love for you will never fade away.

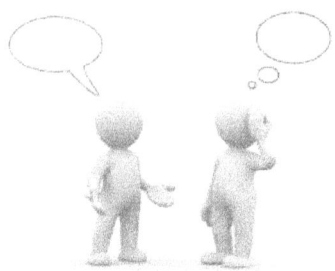

Listen closely, dear one, let it be heard,
Cancer's arrival was never caused by your word.
It's not your fault, please understand,
You are blameless, held in our loving hand.

Listen, my dear, there's something to say,
Cancer has been found, but we won't dismay.
With love as our armor, we'll face each day,
Finding hope and courage along the way.

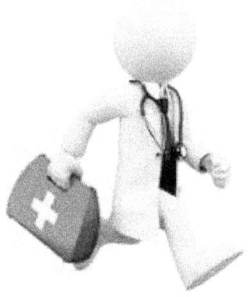

Remember, dear child, you're never alone,
Doctors are here, their expertise shown.
With their support, we'll face cancer's wrath,
And pave the way for a brighter path.

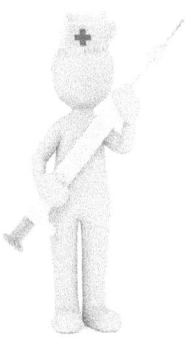

First, there may be blood tests, simple and quick,
To check your health, they'll take just a prick.
They'll look for clues, to understand your fight,
Gathering information, shining a light.

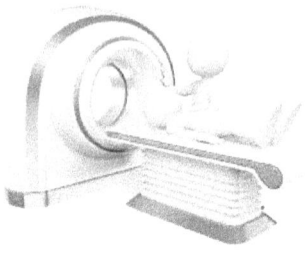

Next, there might be scans, like pictures from afar,
To see inside your body, where the cancer is at par.
You'll lie still, like a superhero at rest,
As the machines capture images, doing their best.

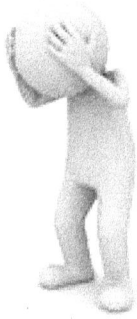

These tests may sound daunting,
but here's what we know,
Each one brings us closer, to help you grow.
The doctors will guide you, every step of the way,
Explaining the process, brightening each day.

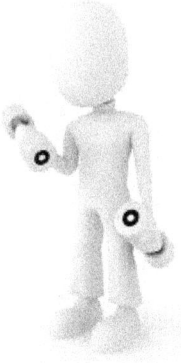

Remember, dear child, you're strong and so brave,
Together we'll face it, one step we'll pave.
These tests are tools, to understand and fight,
With love and support, we'll make things right.

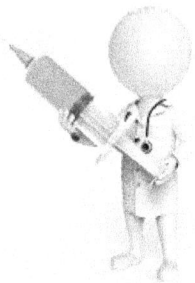

Next, there may be medicines, powerful and strong,
To target the cancer, where it doesn't belong.
They'll fight the battle from deep within,
Attacking the cancer, determined to win.

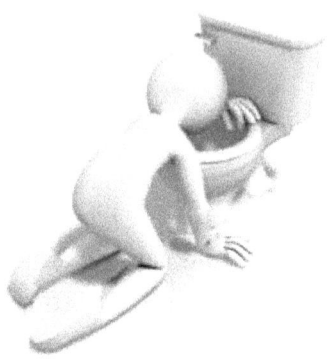

There may be days when energy is low,
And sickness may come and then it may go.
But we'll stand together, through thick and thin,
Supporting you, with love that's akin.

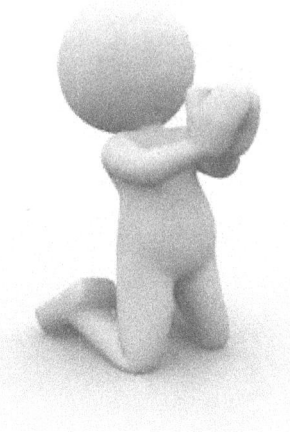

Prayer can bring you comfort, a sense of love and grace,

It connects you to something greater, to a higher place.

Embrace your faith, my precious child, as you stand tall,

Prayer can be a beacon, guiding you through it all.

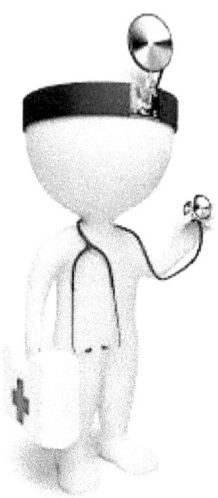

So, trust in these doctors, my courageous one,

With their guidance, the battle will be won.

They'll be by your side, each step of the way,

Helping you fight and brighten each day.

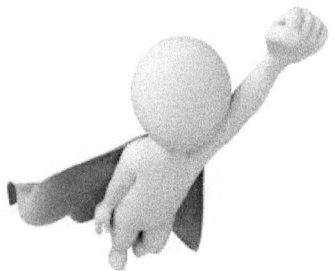

Your superpowers shine, like a beacon in the night,
Inspiring others with your fearless fight.
You face the challenges, with a heart so bold,
A superhero spirit, resilient and untold.

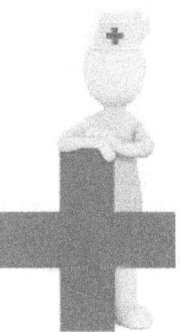

Remember, my brave child, you're incredibly strong,
With each treatment, you're moving along.
The doctors and nurses will guide your flight,
Bringing healing and joy, shining so bright.

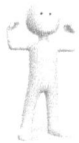

So, trust in the process, and in yourself too,
We'll walk this path, with love all through.
With treatments as our armor, we'll rise above,
Defeating the cancer, with unwavering love.

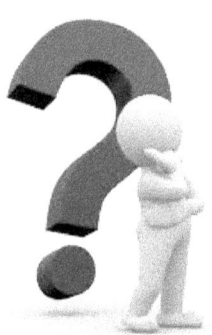

Ask about the treatment, how it will go,
Ask about the doctors, the things they'll show.
Ask about the side effects, what to expect,
Questions are important, they help you connect.

~ 3 ~

WHAT EVERY PARENT SHOULD KNOW

When a parent has a child with cancer, there are several important things to keep in mind. Here are some key points that every parent should know:

Seek specialized medical care: Ensure your child receives treatment from a pediatric oncologist or a specialized cancer center experienced in treating childhood cancers. Pediatric oncologists have the expertise and knowledge to provide the best care for your child.

Understand the diagnosis and treatment plan: Learn as much as you can about your child's diagnosis, including the type of cancer, stage, and treatment options available. Ask questions and communicate openly with the medical team to fully understand the treatment plan, potential side effects, and expected outcomes.

Build a strong support system: Surround yourself with a supportive network of family, friends, and professionals who can offer emotional support, practical assistance, and guidance throughout the journey. Consider joining support groups or connecting with other parents facing similar challenges.

Take care of your own well-being: Caring for a child with cancer can be physically and emotionally draining. It's essential to prioritize self-care, eat healthily, get enough rest, and seek support for your own mental well-being. Taking care of yourself allows you to be better equipped to support your child.

Communicate openly with your child: Be honest and age-appropriate when discussing the diagnosis and treatment with your child. Encourage them to ask questions and express their feelings. Provide reassurance, love, and support while maintaining open lines of communication.

Advocate for your child: Be your child's advocate throughout the treatment process. Ask questions, seek second opinions if needed, and ensure that their needs are met. Stay informed about your child's rights, available resources, and support services.

Take one day at a time: The journey through childhood cancer can be overwhelming. Focus on taking one day at a time and celebrate each milestone and small victory. Lean on your support system and practice self-compassion as you navigate the ups and downs.

Embrace hope and positivity: Cultivate a sense of hope and positivity. While the journey may be challenging, advancements in medical research and treatments provide reason for optimism. Encourage your child to stay positive and find joy amidst the difficulties.

Access available resources: Tap into resources provided by reputable organizations and hospitals specializing in childhood cancer. These resources may include educational materials, financial assistance programs, support groups, and counseling services.

Stay connected with your child's medical team: Maintain open lines of communication with your child's medical team. Attend appointments, ask questions, and keep them informed about any concerns or changes in your child's condition.

They are there to support and guide you throughout the process.

Remember that every child's journey with cancer is unique. It's essential to remain flexible, adapt to changing circumstances, and provide unconditional love and support to your child. Stay hopeful, seek support when needed, and celebrate the strength and resilience of your child and your family.

~ 4 ~

CHILDREN'S NEEDS

Children with cancer have unique needs that go beyond medical treatment. Here are some key aspects to consider:

Emotional support: Children with cancer need emotional support to cope with the challenges they face. They may experience fear, anxiety, and a range of emotions. Providing a nurturing and understanding environment, along with access to mental health professionals and support groups, can make a significant difference.

Normalcy and routine: Maintaining a sense of normalcy and routine is crucial for children with cancer. It helps them feel more secure and provides stability amidst the disruptions caused by medical treatments. Keeping up with schoolwork, engaging in age-appropriate activities, and spending time with friends and siblings can promote a sense of normalcy.

Play and recreation: Play is an essential part of a child's development, even during cancer treatment. It helps them express emotions, relieve stress, and maintain a sense of joy and normalcy. Providing opportunities for play and recreation, whether through toys, games, or creative activities, is important for their overall well-being.

Education and learning: Supporting a child's education and learning during cancer treatment is vital. Ensuring access to educational resources, tutoring, and accommodations can help them stay connected with their studies and provide a sense of continuity in their lives.

Social connections: Children with cancer may experience isolation due to their medical condition. Facilitating social connections and peer support through hospital programs, support groups, or online communities can help combat loneliness and provide a sense of belonging.

Family support: A strong support system is crucial for children with cancer. Providing support to the entire family, including parents and siblings, helps create a nurturing and caring environment. Assistance with practical matters, such as transportation to medical appointments or help with daily tasks, can alleviate some of the burdens faced by the family.

Palliative care and pain management: For children with advanced or terminal cancer, palliative care focuses on providing comfort, pain management, and enhancing quality of life. Access to specialized palliative care services can help alleviate physical and emotional distress for both the child and their family.

Future planning and support: Children with cancer may require assistance in planning for their future, including educational goals, vocational training, and long-term care. Providing guidance and resources to navigate these aspects ensures their well-being beyond their cancer treatment.

Advocacy and awareness: Supporting initiatives that raise awareness about childhood cancer and advocate for research and improved treatments is crucial. Children with cancer benefit from efforts to increase funding, advance scientific knowledge, and improve access to innovative therapies.

Every child's needs are unique, so it's important to communicate openly and listen to their individual preferences and concerns. Collaborating with the child, their family, healthcare professionals, and support organizations can help address their specific needs and provide comprehensive care and support.

~ 5 ~

PARENTS NEEDS

When a child has cancer, parents play a crucial role in supporting their child's well-being. Taking care of themselves is equally important to ensure they have the strength and resilience to be there for their child. Here are some healthy choices parents can consider:

Self-care: Prioritize self-care to maintain physical and mental well-being. This includes getting enough rest, eating a balanced diet, and engaging in activities that promote relaxation and stress reduction, such as exercise, meditation, or pursuing hobbies.

Seek support: Reach out to support networks, such as family, friends, and support groups, for emotional support. Connect with other parents who have gone through a similar experience to share insights and provide mutual support. Consider professional counseling or therapy to cope with the emotional challenges.

Communicate openly: Maintain open and honest communication with the healthcare team about the child's treatment plan, concerns, and any changes in symptoms. Engage in dialogue to fully understand the child's condition and actively participate in decision-making processes.

Educate yourself: Learn about your child's specific type of cancer, treatment options, and potential side effects. This knowledge empowers you to ask informed questions, advocate for your child, and collaborate effectively with the healthcare team.

Organize and manage information: Keep a record of medical appointments, medications, test results, and important contact information. Creating an organized system can help reduce stress, ensure effective communication, and facilitate decision-making.

Maintain a healthy routine: Establish and maintain a regular routine for both yourself and your child. This includes regular meals, consistent sleep patterns, and structured activities. A routine can provide stability and a sense of normalcy during a challenging time.

Engage in physical activity: Incorporate regular exercise into your routine to boost energy levels, reduce stress, and promote overall wellbeing. Find activities that you enjoy and can fit into your schedule, whether it's going for walks, practicing yoga, or engaging in other forms of physical activity.

Practice stress management: Utilize stress management techniques, such as deep breathing exercises, mindfulness, or journaling, to cope with the emotional strain that comes with having a child with cancer. Take breaks when needed and allow yourself time for relaxation and rejuvenation.

Seek respite and support for caregiving: It's essential to ask for help and accept support from family, friends, or community organizations. Allow others to assist with caregiving responsibilities, even if it's for short periods, to recharge and take care of your own needs.

Foster connections: Connect with other parents who have children with cancer. Sharing experiences, advice, and emotions with others who understand can provide comfort and a sense of community.

Remember, taking care of yourself is not selfish but necessary to be a strong source of support for your child. Prioritizing your own well-being will enable you to better navigate the challenges and provide the best possible care for your child with cancer.

~ 6 ~

CHALLENGES

Parents of children with cancer face immense emotional, physical, and practical challenges. Here are some key points to understand about parents of children with cancer:

Emotional impact: Parents experience a wide range of emotions, including shock, fear, sadness, anger, and guilt, upon hearing their child's cancer diagnosis. They may go through periods of intense stress and anxiety as they navigate their child's treatment and well-being.

Caregiving role: Parents become primary caregivers for their child with cancer, often taking on significant responsibilities related to medical appointments, administering medications, managing side effects, coordinating care, and advocating for their child's needs.

Balancing act: Balancing the needs of their child with cancer with the needs of other family members, work, and daily life can be extremely challenging for parents. They often juggle multiple roles and responsibilities, leading to increased stress and exhaustion.

Information and decision-making: Parents must navigate complex medical information, treatment options, and decision-making processes. They may need to make difficult decisions about their child's care, weighing potential risks and benefits while considering their child's best interests.

Financial strain: Childhood cancer treatment can place a significant financial burden on families. Medical expenses, travel costs, accommodation, and other related expenses can quickly accumulate. This financial strain adds an extra layer of stress for parents.

Emotional support: Parents of children with cancer require emotional support to cope with the challenges they face. They benefit from having a strong support network of family, friends, support groups, and mental health professionals who can provide a listening ear, understanding, and empathy.

Self-care and well-being: Parents often neglect their own self-care and well-being while focusing on their child's needs. It's crucial for parents to prioritize their physical and mental health, seek support, and practice self-care to maintain their own resilience and ability to support their child effectively.

Impact on siblings: The experience of having a sibling with cancer can also significantly impact other children in the family. Parents must navigate the emotional needs of their other children and provide support and reassurance during this challenging time.

Advocacy and awareness: Parents of children with cancer often become strong advocates for their child and for childhood cancer awareness. They may engage in advocacy efforts, raise funds for research, and work to raise awareness about childhood cancer and the unique challenges faced by families.

Hope and resilience: Despite the difficulties, parents of children with cancer often demonstrate incredible strength, resilience, and hope. Their unwavering love and commitment to their child's well-being drive them to do whatever it takes to support their child throughout the cancer journey.

Supporting parents of children with cancer involves providing them with emotional support, access to resources, financial assistance, and opportunities to connect with other parents facing similar challenges. Recognizing and honoring their unique experiences and challenges is crucial in helping them navigate this difficult journey with their child.

~ 7 ~

SUPPORT

When a child is diagnosed with cancer, parents face immense challenges and need support to navigate this difficult journey. Here are some key areas where parents of children with cancer can find support:

Medical team communication: Establish open and effective communication with the child's medical team. Ask questions, seek clarification, and actively participate in treatment decisions. Building a strong relationship with healthcare professionals helps ensure the best care for the child.

Local cancer organizations: Research cancer organizations or foundations in your local area that specialize in childhood cancer. They often provide support services, financial assistance, educational resources, and support groups for parents.

Use online directories or search engines to find organizations near you.

Online resources and forums: Explore online resources and forums dedicated to childhood cancer support. Websites and online communities like CancerCare, CaringBridge, or Childhood Cancer Guides offer valuable information, forums for connecting with other parents, and resources specific to the needs of families facing childhood cancer.

National organizations: Reach out to national organizations focused on childhood cancer support, such as the American Childhood Cancer Organization (ACCO), Children's Oncology Group (COG), or St. Jude Children's Research Hospital. They may have resources, helplines, and programs for parents.

Social media groups: Search for social media groups or pages dedicated to childhood cancer support. These communities can provide a platform for sharing experiences, finding emotional support, and connecting with other parents who are going through similar situations.

Local support groups: Check with local hospitals, community centers, or religious organizations for support groups specifically tailored for parents of children with cancer. These groups offer a safe space to share experiences, receive emotional support, and exchange valuable information.

Nonprofit organizations: Look for nonprofit organizations that focus on childhood cancer support. They may offer various resources, financial assistance, counseling services, and programs for parents. Examples include Candlelighters Childhood Cancer Foundation, Alex's Lemonade Stand Foundation, or Ronald McDonald House Charities.

Pediatric oncology clinics or centers: Contact pediatric oncology clinics or treatment centers in your area to inquire about any parent support services they offer. They may have social workers, counselors, or support programs available to provide assistance and guidance.

Recommendations from healthcare professionals: Ask your child's healthcare team for recommendations on local support services and organizations that cater specifically to parents of children with cancer. They may have established relationships with these organizations and can provide valuable insights.

Support networks: Connect with other parents who have children with cancer. Support groups, both in-person and online, provide a space to share experiences, exchange advice, and find comfort in knowing others who understand the journey. Building relationships with these families can offer invaluable support.

Emotional support: Seek emotional support for yourself. Consider joining counseling or therapy sessions to address the complex emotions and stress that come with having a child with cancer. Talking to friends, family, or support organizations can also provide an outlet for sharing concerns and emotions.

Practical support: Accept help from friends, family, and community members. Allow them to assist with practical tasks such as meal preparation, house cleaning, or running errands. Having a support network that can alleviate some of the day-to-day burdens can provide much-needed relief.

Self-care: Prioritize self-care to maintain your own well-being. This includes getting enough rest, eating well, engaging in activities you enjoy, and taking breaks when needed. Taking care of yourself ensures you have the physical and emotional strength to support your child.

Financial assistance: Explore available resources and financial assistance programs. Many organizations provide financial support for medical expenses, transportation costs, and other related needs. Reach out to social workers or financial counselors at the hospital for guidance.

Education and advocacy: Educate yourself about childhood cancer, treatment options, and research advancements. Being informed empowers you to be an advocate for your child and actively participate in their care. Stay updated on the latest developments in pediatric oncology and connect with advocacy organizations.

Siblings' support: Pay attention to the needs of siblings. Their emotions and concerns may sometimes be overshadowed by the child with cancer. Ensure they receive support and maintain open communication with them. Encourage siblings to express their feelings and offer age-appropriate explanations about their sibling's condition.

Respite and self-compassion: Allow yourself breaks and self-compassion. It's normal to feel overwhelmed or exhausted at times. Taking time for self-care, pursuing hobbies, and seeking respite through trusted caregivers or respite programs can help you recharge and maintain your own well-being.

Stay hopeful: Maintain a sense of hope and positivity. Celebrate even small victories and milestones during the treatment process. Cherish moments of joy and focus on the resilience and strength your child exhibits.

Remember, support can come in various forms, including emotional support, financial assistance, educational resources, and connections with other parents who can relate to your experiences. You don't have to face this alone. Reach out for support, advocate for your child, and take care of yourself along the way. The journey may be challenging, but with support and love, you can navigate it together. Don't hesitate to reach out and explore multiple avenues to find the support you need during this challenging time.

~ 8 ~

RESOURCES

Parents of children with cancer can benefit from a wide range of resources tailored to their unique needs. Here are some valuable resources to consider:

American Childhood Cancer Organization (ACCO): ACCO provides comprehensive resources and support for families facing childhood cancer. Their website offers information about different types of childhood cancers, treatment options, coping strategies, and access to support services.

Children's Oncology Group (COG): COG is the world's largest organization dedicated to childhood cancer research. Their website provides resources for families, including treatment guidelines, clinical trials information, and educational materials.

National Cancer Institute (NCI): NCI offers a dedicated section on childhood cancers on their website, providing information about different types of childhood cancers, treatment options, clinical trials, and supportive care resources.

St. Jude Children's Research Hospital: St. Jude provides extensive resources for families, including information about childhood cancers, treatment protocols, educational materials, and supportive care resources. They also offer support services and resources for parents and siblings.

CureSearch for Children's Cancer: CureSearch offers resources and educational materials for parents, including information about childhood cancers, treatment options, clinical trials, and coping strategies. They also provide support services and access to research updates.

National Children's Cancer Society (NCCS): NCCS offers various resources and support programs for families, including financial assistance, emotional support services, educational resources, and advocacy initiatives.

Pediatric Oncology Resource Center (PORC): PORC provides a wealth of information and resources for parents, including educational materials, support group listings, financial assistance resources, and information about psychosocial support services.

CancerCare: CancerCare offers free support services for individuals and families affected by cancer. They provide counseling services, support groups, educational resources, financial assistance programs, and online forums for parents of children with cancer.

Alex's Lemonade Stand Foundation: Alex's Lemonade Stand Foundation offers resources and support for families of children with cancer. They provide information about childhood cancers, research updates, financial assistance programs, and support services.

Local hospitals and clinics: Contact your local pediatric oncology hospitals or clinics to inquire about resources and support programs available to parents. They may have social workers, support groups, educational materials, and other resources tailored to the needs of parents of children with cancer.

Remember to also reach out to your child's healthcare team, as they can provide guidance, recommendations, and additional resources specific to your child's diagnosis and treatment.

~ 9 ~

AGENCIES

There are various agencies and organizations that provide support specifically for parents of children with cancer. Here are some notable agency resources:

Family Support America: Family Support America connects families to local agencies and support services. They offer a directory of family support programs across the United States, including those focused on childhood cancer support.

Ronald McDonald House Charities (RMHC): RMHC provides accommodation and support services to families of seriously ill children. Their Ronald McDonald Houses offer a "home away from home" for families while their child receives treatment. They also provide family rooms within hospitals, scholarships, and other resources.

Social Security Administration (SSA): The SSA offers support programs, including Supplemental Security Income (SSI) and Social Security Disability Insurance (SSDI), which provide financial assistance to families of children with disabilities, including those with cancer.

Make-A-Wish Foundation: Make-A-Wish grants the wishes of children with critical illnesses, including cancer. They provide support and memorable experiences to bring joy and hope to children and their families.

National Children's Cancer Society (NCCS): NCCS offers support services for families affected by childhood cancer. Their programs include financial assistance, emotional support, educational resources, advocacy, and information on survivorship issues.

Be the Match: Be the Match is a registry of potential bone marrow and stem cell donors. They assist families in finding potential matches and provide support throughout the transplant process.

Children's Cancer Association (CCA): CCA offers support programs and resources for families of children with cancer. Their programs include Chemo Pal Mentoring, Music Rx, and the Alexandra

Ellis Caring Cabin, which provides retreats for families to relax and reconnect.

Candlelighters Childhood Cancer Foundation: Candlelighters provides support services, including financial assistance, educational resources, and emotional support, to families of children with cancer. They have chapters across the United States offering local support.

National Organization for Rare Disorders (NORD): NORD offers resources and support for families of children with rare forms of cancer. They provide information, advocacy, and connections to specialized support groups and clinical trials.

Local and regional cancer organizations: Many local and regional cancer organizations offer support programs and resources for families. These organizations often provide financial assistance, counseling services, support groups, and educational materials specific to the community they serve.

It's important to research and reach out to these agencies to explore the specific support services they offer and how they can assist you and your family. Additionally, your child's healthcare team or social workers at the hospital may also be able to provide recommendations and connect you with local agency resources.

~ 10 ~

MY CHILDHOOD EXPERIENCE

I was 9 years old when I was told I had cancer and that is why I'm sharing my experience. For me, I thought I was unique and different but that isn't true. All I can do is provide some insight on my treatments, side effects, test, and my miracle outcome. But note, the journey is different for each patient and their family but this is meant to give you hope.

In early Spring of 1978, I became ill. It started with having flu like symptoms during the night, but in the morning, I felt great and wanted to go to school. Being an only child, school is a needed social outlet and I had FOMO - fear of missing out. Then all sudden, I started to get sick during the day at school. I would have to be sent home and mom was encouraged to take me to my doctor to be seen.

My family doctor, Dr. Melvin Dyster, was a great doctor. He was the only doctor I knew. We were able to get in quick with Dr. Dyster. I felt abdominal pain accompanied with mild fever. I was admitted to Niagara Falls Memorial Hospital and treated under the impression of Crohn's disease with partial obstruction. I was treated with Prednisone and oxazolidine without improvement. So, I was transferred to Buffalo Children's Hospital; I got to ride in an ambulance.

Arrived and admitted to Buffalo Children's Hospital on 3-10-78. While at Children's Hospital, I began to get much worse. Test after test still provided no insight on what was going on. Later investigations showed an abdominal mass in the right lower quadrant with bilateral pleural effusion. I had exploratory laparotomy, which was done 4-3-78. Biopsy revealed mass to Burkitt's Lymphoma Stag IV. Burkitt's lymphoma is quite rare outside of Africa. Since Burkitt's lymphoma has the highest growth rate of any tumor in man, rapid diagnosis and immediate treatment are important and likely to improve outcome.

I developed a uric acid nephropathy and was treated with chemotherapy with Cytoxan, 2 doses, 130mg, and one dose of Vincristine. Uric acid nephropathy, is a series of kidney disorders caused by an increase in uric acid in the human serum, All Buffalo Children's Hospital could do for me was quality of life treatment until my passing. Given the severity of the case and grim prognosis, I was given less than one year to live. Dr. Green, a consultant from Roswell Park Memorial Hospital, reviewed my case and believed they could do something for me. He spoke to my mother, and me, explaining how they had very aggressive treatment plan; High-dose cyclophosphamide and intermediate-dose methotrexate for the treatment of far-advanced Burkitt's lymphoma.

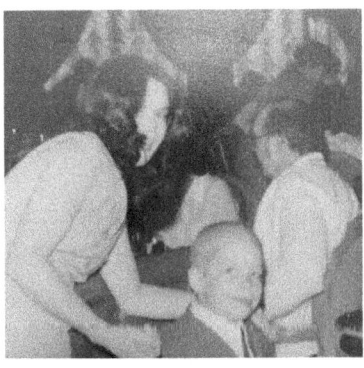

This me on my tenth birthday...

Some of the treatment plans/medications were still in experimental phase. But Dr. Green believed that they could increase my survivability rate by 25%, but I could also die from complications within three months. My mother, with zero support and at the age of 26 years old, I was 9, had to make a life or death decision and risking I could die sooner. It was an easy decision for my mother, stay at Children's and die within a year or take a chance and have a 25% survivability outcome.

I was transferred and admitted to Roswell Park Memorial Institute on 4-10-78 at the age of nine years and ten months, with history of an abdominal mass with vomiting for a few weeks prior to admission. I noted abdominal swelling for almost nine months prior to admission. Six weeks prior to admission, I felt abdominal pain accompanied with mild fever.

Roswell Park Memorial, then changed to Roswell Park Cancer Institute, and now is call Roswell Park Comprehensive Cancer Center, was America's first cancer center, founded in 1898 by Dr. Roswell Park in Buffalo, New York. His revolutionary model of a "multidisciplinary approach" to cancer — with scientists and clinicians working in concert and in consult — has become the standard by which all modern-day comprehensive.

I was admitted to the hospital and treated with chemotherapy in the following regimen. He received Vincristine, Cytoxan, Prednisone, and intrathecal Methotrexate.

> Vincristine is a chemotherapy drug that belongs to a group of drugs called vinca alkaloids. Vincristine works by stopping the cancer cells from separating into 2 new cells. So, it stops the growth of the cancer.

> Cyclophosphamide is a chemotherapy medication that slows the growth of cancer cells. It treats lymphoma, myeloma, leukemia, breast cancer and

ovarian cancer. When I was receiving this med, it was given IV push. I became part of an experimental group to try it in tablet form. It is now given in a tablet form that you can take by mouth with a glass of water. The brand name of this medication is Cytoxan®.

Prednisone is approved use to treat nausea and vomiting associated with some chemotherapy drugs. Used to stimulate appetite in cancer patients with severe appetite problems. Also used to replace steroids in conditions of adrenal insufficiency (low production of needed steroids produced by the adrenal glands).

Methotrexate sodium is a type of chemotherapy called an antimetabolite. Methotrexate sodium kills cancer cells by preventing them from making DNA. Methotrexate sodium may also help the body's immune system kill the cancer.

The day after receiving his first dose of Cytoxan, he was taken to the operating room to and multiple aspirates of bone marrow were obtained. I received I.V. Methotrexate and intrathecal Methotrexate on 5-14-78. Five days later, the bone marrow, which was removed, was replaced back into me. One of Roswell Parks first successful pediatric bone marrow transplants using the patient's own barrow.

My blood counts after intensive therapy became quite low with WBC reaching a nadir of 200 and platelet count reaching a nadir of 11,000 on 5-18-78. Nadir means lowest point. The normal number of WBCs in the blood is 4,500 to 11,000. A normal platelet count ranges from 150,000 to 450,000. I was put into isolation to protect me from outside germs, viruses, and diseases. I did however get a Lysing infection in my left index finger, secondary to fingerstick blood draw. It was scary at the time, everyone having fully grown up from head to toe to come in and see me. Only essential staff could enter; I could see my mom from the room window that looked out onto the hallway.

After getting my blood levels to an acceptable rate, they eased up on the isolation protocols. Unfortunately, I spiked high temperatures and was treated IV antibiotics. Then I developed a hemorrhagic cystitis with blood passing in my urine after high-dose Cytoxan. This was treated with high volume of IV fluids and cleared up.

Later after that, from all the treatments, I developed oral Methotrexate lesions, which were very painful. Inflammation of the lining of the mouth (mucositis) which can lead to oral ulceration is a possible side-effect of methotrexate, especially if methotrexate is taken in high doses (such as in cancer treatment). Patients can experience mouth ulcers, which I did. This too resolved over time and with treatment. Testing was countless: bloodwork, fingerstick, CT scans, ultrasounds, gallium scans, born marrow aspirations, spinal taps, upper and lower GI, and x-rays. But all of it was worth it because, on June 5, 2023, I turned 55, and I'm doing pretty good if I say so myself.

There has been studies done that indicate a high probability of Posttraumatic Stress Disorder in Adult Survivors of Childhood Cancer. I know that I have experiences this and use to have nightmares leading up to any of my follow-up appointments associated with my cancer. To this day, I can't stand going to the doctors. When I have test done, I worry until the results come in. Sometimes this has incapacitated me to where I am unable to think of anything else or do anything. Always a fear of hearing those words, "You have cancer."

www.ingramcontent.com/pod-product-compliance
Lightning Source LLC
Chambersburg PA
CBHW070035040426
42333CB00040B/1685